Complete
Renal Diet
Cookbook

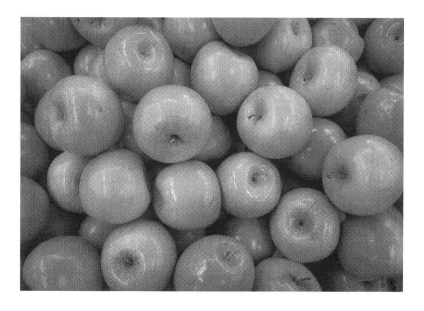

THE OPTIMAL RECIPE BOOK TO MANAGE KIDNEY DISEASE AND AVOID DIALYSIS!

Table of Contents

Introduction

Have you been diagnosed with renal disease? If yes, and your doctor has advised you some general diet guidelines on what to eat and what to avoid, may be you still wondering about some details and recipes to try out while being on a renal diet.

Being in the first stages of renal damage you should follow Renal diet correctly as it can slow down the progression of the disease and help you avoid dialysis.

In this book, we aim to tackle all your main concerns regarding renal diet and give you detailed recipes that follow all renal diet specifics, so keep on reading...

What is Kidney Disease? Main Causes.

Kidney disease or in other worlds "renal disease" and "kidney damage" is a health condition where the kidneys are unable to function in a healthy and proper manner.

How kidneys work and what is their role in our systems?

Kidneys are vital organs located in our lower body backs (around the ribcage area) that are responsible for filtering out the toxins and junk out of our bloodstream through the urine. To preserve the balance in our systems, kidneys help regulate salts and minerals circulating in our bodies such as sodium, phosphorus, and potassium. Our kidneys also release hormonal compounds that help regulate blood pressure, build new red blood cells, and maintain the health of bones and connective tissue.

Kidney disease, in this case, is a chronic condition (CKD) where the kidneys fail gradually to do their normal job. Chronic kidney disease typically develops in 5 stages. Each stage is measured by a formula called Glomerular Filtration Rate (GFR) which is calculated by several variables like age, race, gender, and the amount of serum creatinine in the urine. The higher this protein is in the system, the more progressed the stage of renal disease will be. Here is a brief snapshot of each stage.

Stage 1: considered normal or high risk of developing CKD. The GFR falls > 90 mL/min.

Stage 2: considered as mild CKD. The GFR falls in the range of 60-89 mL/min.

Stage 3: Moderate CKD which ranges from 45-59 mL/min.

Stage 4: Severe Chronic Kidney disease. Rates fall between 15-29 mL/min.

Stage 5: Final/end stage of renal disease which calls for surgery or dialysis. Also known as End Stage Renal Disease (ESRD). The GFR levels, in this case, fall below 15 mL/min.

Now in regards to the actual causes or risk factors that may contribute to the formation of disease, studies have indicated the following conditions:

Diabetes. Diabetes is probably the No.1 cause of renal disease as the increased blood glucose in the bloodstream can actually ruin blood vessels inside the kidneys.

Heart disease. Heart disease has also been found to have a negative association with CKD. Those with chronic heart problems, in particular, have a higher probability of developing renal disease as well.

Elevated blood pressure. Abnormally high blood pressure, similarly to diabetes can ruin the delicate blood vessels inside the kidneys and make them function poorly as a result.

Genetic History of Renal Disease. If any of your family members and especially parents and grandparents have already developed the disease, there is a higher risk you are going to develop it too. If any of your family members has kidney disease, it would be wise to get tested too and encourage other family members to do the same.

In addition to the above common causes, autoimmune disorders like Lupus and nephrotic syndrome can increase the risk of developing renal disease. Also, urinary problems and certain medications e.g. diuretics or antibiotics, as well as illegal drugs, can also interfere with the normal function of the kidneys and cause damage. For this reason, it would be wise to consult your doctor and take drugs for other conditions e.g. diabetes that does not harm your kidneys as a side effect.

The problem with the disease is that it often comes with little or no symptoms at all, especially during the first stages. You may experience the following symptoms, but these could also be a sign of another condition:

- Less frequent urination
- Very little amount of urine
- Sudden and unexplained pauses in breath
- Nausea
- Chest or back pain
- Drowsiness and dizziness
- Fatigue/feeling tired more than before
- Confusion
- Loss of balance
- Swelling in the face, ankles, feet, and hands
- Poor appetite

In extreme cases and stages e.g. renal failure, seizures and coma may also occur. However, it would be best for you to avoid looking solely for these symptoms and actually get tested to find out whether you have a chronic disease or not.

The History of Renal Diet

A renal diet is a medical treatment measure that has been followed for over three decades to stop the progression of renal disease. The vast majority of doctors and hospitals advise their patients to follow a renal diet program for this purpose.

Along with certain prescribed medications and lifestyle changes, renal disease has been proven to be a valuable weapon against the need for hemodialysis.

Why do You Need Renal Diet?

Renal typically based on certain foods that are low in sodium, potassium, and phosphorus, which are minerals that are known to help build up fluid in the system. When you have renal disease though, these fluids cannot be easily expelled by your kidneys through the urine and so you must limit their consumption so that there is no risk of fluid build-up and worsening of the disease.

Renal diet, in general decreases the likelihood of renal disorder progression through the following ways:

- Minimizes risky fluid build up from high levels of minerals, as the kidneys cannot process excessive amounts on their own.

- Encourages the consumption of high-quality protein, while limiting the amount of bad protein that could be damaging to the kidneys.

- Helps keep the minerals, electrolytes, and salts in our system balanced partially replacing your kidneys function when they can't fully work on their own.

A renal diet is especially useful during stages 1-3 as it is mainly used as a preventive measure rather than an actual treatment for patients in more advanced renal disease stages. However, if you follow the diet and a healthy lifestyle, there is a very high chance to avoid dialysis and live a quality life.

The Explanation of Key Diet Words

When following a renal diet, certain nutrients are very important as they can actually make worse or improve chronic kidney disorder. Here is a brief list of the most important ones

Potassium.

Potassium is a naturally occurring mineral found in nearly all foods, in varying amounts. Our bodies need an amount of potassium to help with muscle activity as well as electrolyte balance and regulation of blood pressure. However, when there is an excessive amount of potassium in the system and the kidneys can't expel it (due to renal disease), fluid retention and muscle spasms can occur.

Phosphorus.

Phosphorus is a trace mineral found in a wide range of foods and especially dairy, meat, and eggs. It acts synergistically with calcium as well as Vitamin D to promote bone health. However, when there is damage in the kidneys, excess amounts of the mineral cannot be taken out and this can cause bone weakness.

Calories.

When being on a renal diet, it is important to give yourself the right amount of calories to fuel your system. The exact amount of calories you should consume daily depends on your age, gender, general health status and stage of renal disease. In most cases though, there are no strict limitations in the calorie intake, as long as you take them from proper sources that are low in sodium, potassium, and phosphorus. In general, doctors recommend a daily limit between 1800-2100 calories per day to keep weight within the normal range.

Protein.

Protein is an essential nutrient that our systems need to develop and generate new connective tissue e.g. muscles, even during injuries. Protein also helps stop bleeding and helps the immune system fight infections. A healthy adult with no kidney disease would normally need 40-65 grams of protein per day.

However, in renal diet, protein consumption is a tricky subject as too much or too little can cause problems. Protein, when being metabolized by our systems also creates waste which is typically processed by the kidneys. But when kidneys are damaged or underperforming, as in the case of kidney disease that waste will stay in the system. This is why patients in more advanced CKD stages, are advised to limit their protein consumption as well.

Fats.

Fats and particularly good fats are needed by our systems as a fuel source and for other metabolic cell functions. A diet rich in bad and trans or saturated fats though can greatly raise the odds of developing heart problems, which often occur with renal disease. This is why most physicians advise their renal patients to follow a diet that contains a decent amount of good fats and a very low amount of trans (processed) or saturated fat.

Sodium.

Sodium is an essential mineral that our bodies need to regulate fluid and electrolyte balance. It also plays a role in normal cell division in the muscles and nervous system. However, in kidney disease, sodium can quickly spike at higher than normal levels and the kidneys will be unable to expel it causing fluid accumulation as a side-effect. Those who also suffer from heart problems as well should limit its consumption as it may raise blood pressure.

Carbohydrates.

Carbs act as a major and quick fuel source for the body's cells. When we consume carbs, our systems turn them into glucose and then into energy for "feeding" our body cells. Carbs are generally not restricted in renal diet but some types of carbs contain dietary fiber as well, which helps regulate normal colon function and protect blood vessels from damage.

Dietary Fiber.

Fiber is an important element in our system that cannot be properly digested but plays a key role in the regulation of our bowel movements and blood cell protection. The fiber in the renal diet is generally encouraged as it helps loosen up the stools, relieve constipation and bloating and protect from colon damage. However, many patients don't get enough amounts of dietary fiber per day as many of them are high in potassium or phosphorus. Fortunately, there are some good dietary fiber sources for CKD patients that have lower amounts of these minerals compared to others.

Vitamins/Minerals.

Our systems, according to medical research, need at least 13 vitamins and minerals to keep our cells fully active and healthy. Patients with renal disease though are more likely to be depleted by water-soluble vitamins like Bcomplex and Vitamin C, as a result, or limited fluid consumption. Therefore, supplementation with these vitamins along with a renal diet program should help cover any possible vitamin deficiencies. Supplementation of fat-soluble vitamins like vitamins A, K, and E may be avoided as they can quickly build up in the system and turn toxic.

Fluids.

When you are in an advanced stage of renal disease, fluid can quickly build-up and lead to problems. While it is important to keep your system well hydrated, you should avoid minerals like potassium and sodium which can trigger further fluid build-up and cause a host of other symptoms.

What Food to Eat and What to Avoid?

Being on a renal diet, you are probably wondering which foods you can consume and which you can avoid. As it was specified earlier, you need to consume foods that are naturally low in sodium, potassium, and phosphorus. These foods are:

- Red forest fruits e.g. berries, blueberries, strawberries, raspberries
- Red bell peppers
- Corn
- Cabbage
- Lettuce
- Broccoli
- Cauliflower
- Garlic
- Onions
- Celery
- Apples

- Cherries
- Red Grapes
- Peaches
- Figs
- Egg whites
- Vegetable oils e.g. olive oil or safflower oil
- Soy milk
- Egg whites
- Cream cheese
- Cottage cheese
- Parmesan cheese
- Fresh fish and seafood e.g. mahi-mahi tuna, lobster, crab, oysters, and shrimp
- Imitation fish e.g. crab sticks
- Pasta
- Bread
- Unfortified rice milk
- Corn cereals
- Green beans
- Radishes

- Beef (in moderate amounts)
- Turkey
- Chicken

Make sure that you eat fresh and unprocessed versions of the above as dried fruits or canned fish and meat may be possibly loaded with hidden amounts of extra sodium and phosphorus.

Now, when it comes to foods that you should avoid, although you don't have to avoid them completely for long periods of time, it's best to limit their consumption as they contain high amounts of sodium, phosphorus and/or potassium:

- Avocadoes
- Bananas
- Lentils
- Beans
- Spinach
- Swiss chard

- Mature cheeses e.g. cheddar or gouda
- Cow milk
- Most dairy products
- Liver and organ meats
- Brewer's yeast
- Egg yolks
- Chocolate
- Cola's
- Custard
- Dairy ice-cream
- Potatoes
- Oranges
- Apricots
- Dried fruit
- Pickles and relish
- Packaged crisps and crackers
- Brown rice
- Most packed and canned food e.g. cream soups or spam.

Be extra cautious as phosphorus can cleverly hide in many packed food labels, under different chemical names such as:

- Phosphoric acid
- Disodium phosphate
- Monosodium phosphate
- Trisodium phosphate
- Dicalcium phosphate
- Tetrasodium pyrophosphate

If you notice any of the above names in the top 5 ingredients of a food label, it typically means that the food is high in phosphorus and should be avoided.

List of Juices and Drinks in Renal Diet

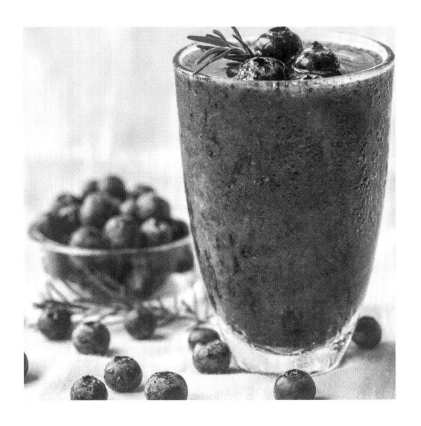

When following a renal diet, keeping yourself hydrated without exceeding the liquid limit of 2.5 liters per day is very important. If you are currently at a more progressed stage e.g. stage 4, your doctor may suggest you limit the consumption of fluids up to 2 liters per day. In most cases, you can drink:

- Plain or fruit-infused water
- Homemade ice tea
- Grape juice
- Berry juice
- Peach juice
- Green tea
- Caffeine-free herbal tea e.g. chamomile.
- Almond milk
- Soda water
- Lemonade
- Light colored fizzy drinks e.g. sprite
- Coffee in moderate amounts
- Coffee alternatives with fig and chicory wood.
- Low-fat goat milk
- Smoothies with berries, peaches, apples or celery blended with water or almond milk.

You may also consume low alcoholic drinks like wine and beer in moderate amounts and preferably not more than 5 cups per week.

Frequently Asked Questions

Q: How can I figure out if a food label or recipe is low in potassium and what is the maximum daily limit?

A: When following a renal diet, you ideally want to make sure that potassium levels are below 250mg/per serving or up to 7% of the food's total nutritional value. If the food/recipe indicates less than 100 mg of potassium per serving, this means that it's very low in potassium, however, a moderate rate of up to 250 mg per serving is fine, as long as you don't consume any other foods throughout the day with moderate or high potassium levels e.g. between 250-400 mg/serving.

Q: Is it possible to lose weight during a renal diet?

A: If you wish to lose extra weight for health or fitness reasons, you can follow a renal diet plan that is preferably high in fats and fiber foods e.g. forest fruits, cabbage, etc. You still want to make sure that your daily calorie intake does not exceed 2000 calories and any foods that you choose are low in sodium and potassium to keep bloating and fluid build-up under control. The exact amount of calories that you need to take though, depends on your age, gender, health status and the weight goal that you wish to achieve. If you wish to lose weight as well with your renal diet plan, it's better to discuss the matter with an expert dietician or nutritionist.

Q: Does my CKD stage count when following a renal diet?

A: Absolutely! In earlier stages (up to the third stage), it is fine to consume low to moderate amounts of sodium, potassium, and phosphorus while your fluid intake should be up to 2.5 liters per day. However, when you are in a more advanced stage of renal damage, you have to limit all the above minerals and fluids further e.g. drink up to 2 liters of fluids per day or only up to 150 mg of potassium per meal (instead of 250mg). Your doctor or dietician will give you additional guidelines on the exact amounts of each that you need to take daily, based on your current stage of renal disease.

Q: Is it OK to take caffeine in a renal diet?

A: In most cases and especially during the first three stages of CKD, a caffeine-based drink is perfectly fine. You may drink up to 2 cups of coffee or caffeine tea per day without any worries. However, be careful as any extras that you add to your coffee will not only increase calories, they may raise potassium levels as well. Such toppings are whipping cream, caramel syrups, chocolate, etc. Pure coffee or black tea with water and a bit of almond or soy milk isn't an issue but anything "fortified" should be avoided.

Q: Can I take over the counter medication when on a renal diet?

A: Unfortunately, the vast majority of over the counter medication/painkillers like aspirin and ibuprofen are not indicated for CKD patients. Any drug that belongs in the NSAID (nonsteroidal anti-inflammatory drugs) category should be avoided as according to some studies, NSAIDs can worsen CKD. Some other types of medication are also not indicated for renal patients. If you are currently taking any other medication, it would be wise to consult your doctor to find out whether they are OK for kidney function or not.

Recipes

Breakfast

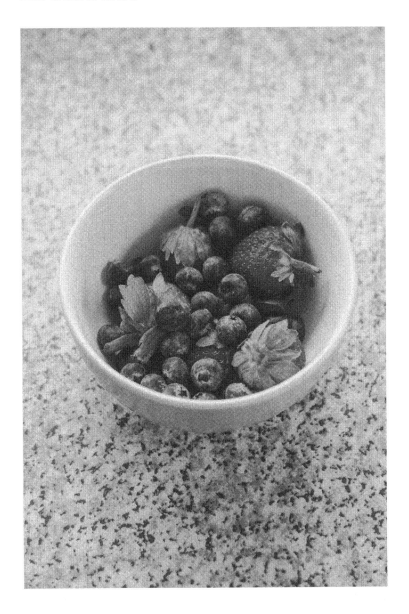

Egg White and Pepper Omelette

COOKING TIME: 5 MIN

DESCRIPTION

A low-calorie omelette recipe with red bell peppers that you can make in under 5 minutes with just 5 ingredients. Feel free to enhance its taste with paprika or Mexican spices.

INGREDIENTS FOR 1-2 SERVINGS

- 4 egg whites, lightly beaten
- 1 red bell pepper, diced
- 1 tsp of paprika
- 2 tbsp of olive oil
- ½ tsp of salt
- Pepper

METHOD

1. In a shallow pan (around 8 inches), heat the olive oil and saute the bell peppers until softened.

2. Add the egg whites and the paprika and fold the edges into the fluid center with a spatula and let omelette cook until eggs are fully opaque and solid.
3. Season with salt and pepper.
4. Serve.

NUTRITIONAL INFORMATION (Per Serving)

- Calories: 165 kcal
- Carbohydrate: 3.8 g
- Protein: 9.2 g
- Sodium: 797 mg
- Potassium: 193 mg
- Phosphorus: 202.5 mg
- Dietary Fiber: 0.7 g
- Fat: 15.22 g

Blueberry Smoothie Bowl

COOKING TIME: 1 MIN

DESCRIPTION

An Instagram worthy purple smoothie bowl made with frozen blueberries that are fortified with antioxidants. Plus, it counts less than 150 mg of potassium and phosphorus per serving.

INGREDIENTS FOR 1 SERVING

- ½ cup of frozen blueberries
- ½ cup of vanilla flavored almond milk
- 1 tbsp of agave syrup
- 1 tsp of chia seeds

METHOD

1. Combine everything except for the chia seeds in the blender until smooth. You should end up with a thick smoothie paste.

2. Transfer into a cereal bowl and top with chia seeds on top.

NUTRITIONAL INFORMATION (Per Serving)

- Calories: 278.5 kcal
- Carbohydrate: 38.72 g
- Protein: 1.3 g
- Sodium: 76.33 mg
- Potassium: 229.1 mg
- Phosphorus: 59.2 mg
- Dietary Fiber: 7.4 g
- Fat: 6 g

Turkey Breakfast Sausage

COOKING TIME: 6 MIN

DESCRIPTION

Fancy a quick sausage for breakfast or brunch? Try this low potassium breakfast sausage with turkey and spices-feel free to serve this with cornbread and apple sauce.

INGREDIENTS FOR 12 SERVINGS

(12 patties per recipe)

- 1 pound of lean ground turkey
- 1 tsp of fennel seed
- ¼ tsp garlic powder
- ¼ tsp onion powder
- ¼ tsp salt
- 2 tbsp of vegetable oil
- Pepper

METHOD

1. Combine all the ingredients apart from the vegetable oil in a mixing bowl.
2. Form into long and flat (around 4 inch-long) patties.
3. Heat the vegetable oil in a medium frying pan.
4. Add 3-4 patties at a time and cook for approx. 3 minutes on each side. Repeat until you cook all patties.
5. Serve warm.

NUTRITIONAL INFORMATION (Per Serving)

- Calories: 74 kcal
- Carbohydrate: 0.1 g
- Protein: 7 g
- Sodium: 121.9 mg
- Potassium: 89.5 mg
- Phosphorus: 75 mg
- Dietary Fiber: 0 g
- Fat: 5.16 g

Italian Apple Fritters

COOKING TIME: 8 MIN

DESCRIPTION

A quick apple fritter recipe with corn flour batter that is great for breakfast and dessert too. Make this preferably in a deep fryer and enjoy hot as it will lose its crisp after a few minutes.

INGREDIENTS FOR 4 SERVINGS

- 2 large apples, seeded, peeled and thickly sliced in round circles
- 3 tbsp of corn flour
- ½ tsp of water
- 1 tsp of sugar
- 1 tsp of cinnamon
- Vegetable oil (for frying)
- Sprinkle of icing sugar or honey

METHOD

1. In a small bowl, combine the corn flour, water and sugar to make your batter
2. Deep the apple rounds into the cornflour mix.
3. Heat enough vegetable oil to cover half of the pan's surface over medium to high heat.
4. Add the apple rounds into the pan and cook until golden brown.
5. Transfer into a shallow dish with absorbing paper on top and sprinkle with a bit of cinnamon and icing sugar.

NUTRITIONAL INFORMATION (Per Serving)

- Calories: 183 kcal
- Carbohydrate: 17.9 g
- Protein: 0.3 g
- Sodium: 2 g
- Potassium: 100 mg
- Phosphorus: 12.5 mg
- Dietary Fiber: 1.4 g
- Fat: 14.17 g

Tofu and Mushroom Scramble

COOKING TIME: 7-8 MIN

DESCRIPTION

A hearty mushroom scramble recipe for vegans or fans of earthy mushroom flavors enhanced by a fine blend of exotic spices. Great for breakfast or a delicious savory brunch.

INGREDIENTS FOR 2 SERVINGS

- ½ cup of sliced white mushrooms
- ⅓ cup medium firm tofu, crumbled
- 1 tbsp of chopped shallots
- ⅓ tsp turmeric
- 1 tsp of cumin
- ⅓ tsp of smoked paprika
- ½ tsp of garlic salt
- Pepper
- 3 tbsp of vegetable oil

METHOD

1. Heat the oil in a medium frying pan and saute the sliced mushrooms with the shallots until softened (around 3-4 minutes) over medium to high heat.
2. Add the tofu pieces and toss in the spices and the garlic salt. Toss lightly until tofu and mushrooms are nicely combined together.
3. Serve warm.

NUTRITIONAL INFORMATION (Per Serving)

- Calories: 220 kcal
- Carbohydrate: 2.59 g
- Protein: 3.2 g
- Sodium: 288 mg
- Potassium: 133.5 mg
- Phosphorus: 68.5 mg
- Dietary Fiber: 1.7 g
- Fat: 23.7 g

Sunny Pineapple Breakfast Smoothie

COOKING TIME: 1 MIN

DESCRIPTION

A sunny and bright breakfast smoothie with the sweet and sour goodness of pineapple blended with a hint of ginger for that zingy fresh taste.

INGREDIENTS FOR 1 SERVING.

- ½ cup of frozen pineapple chunks
- ⅔ cup almond milk
- ½ tsp of ginger powder
- 1 tbsp of agave syrup

METHOD

1. Blend everything together in a blender until nice and smooth (around 30 seconds).
2. Transfer into a tall glass or mason jar.

NUTRITIONAL INFORMATION (Per Serving)

- Calories: 186 kcal
- Carbohydrate: 43.7 g
- Protein: 2.28 g
- Sodium: 130 mg
- Potassium: 135 mg
- Phosphorus: 18 mg
- Dietary Fiber: 2.4 g
- Fat: 2.3 g

Puff Oven Pancakes

COOKING TIME: 30 MIN

DESCRIPTION

A crunchy oven pancake recipe with rice flour that is very low in potassium and phosphorus. Try this if you want something crunchy and interesting compared to ordinary pancakes.

INGREDIENTS FOR 4 SERVINGS

- 2 large eggs.
- ½ cup of rice flour
- ½ cup of rice milk
- 2 tbsp of unsalted butter
- ⅛ tsp salt

METHOD

1. Preheat the oven at 400F/190C.
2. Grease a 10-inch skillet or Pyrex with the butter and heat in the oven until it melts.

3. In a mixing bowl, beat the eggs and whisk in the rice milk, flour and salt until smooth.
4. Take off the skillet or pie dish from the oven.
5. Transfer directly the batter into the skillet and put back in the oven for 25-30 minutes.
6. Place in a serving dish and cut into 4 portions.
7. Serve hot with honey or icing sugar on top.

NUTRITIONAL INFORMATION (Per Serving)

- Calories: 159.75 kcal
- Carbohydrate: 17 g
- Protein: 5 g
- Sodium: 120 g
- Potassium: 52 mg
- Phosphorus: 66.25 mg
- Dietary Fiber: 0.5 g
- Fat: 9 g

Savory Muffins with Protein

COOKING TIME 35 MIN

DESCRIPTION

A great alternative to sweet and tangy blueberry muffins. This savory muffin recipe is great alone or as a part of your breakfast. You can take it with some bacon or homemade sausage on the side and it will be delicious.

INGREDIENTS FOR 12 SERVINGS

- 2 cups of corn flakes
- ½ cup of unfortified almond milk
- 4 large eggs
- 2 tbsp of olive oil
- 1/2 cup of almond milk
- 1 medium white onion, sliced
- 1 cup of plain Greek yogurt
- ¼ cup pecans, chopped
- 1 tbsp of mixed seasoning blend e.g. Mrs. dash

METHOD

1. Preheat the oven at 350F/180C.
2. Heat the olive oil in the pan. Saute the onions with the pecans and seasoning blend for a couple of minutes.
3. Add the rest of ingredients and toss well.
4. Split the mixture into 12 small muffin cups (lightly greased) and bake for 30-35 minutes or until an inserted knife or toothpick is coming out clean.
5. Serve warm or keep at room temperature for a couple of days.

NUTRITIONAL INFORMATION (Per Serving)

- Calories: 106.58 kcal
- Carbohydrate: 8.20 g
- Protein: 4.77 g
- Sodium: 51.91 mg
- Potassium: 87.83 mg
- Phosphorus: 49.41 mg
- Dietary Fiber: 0.58 g
- Fat: 5 g

Tex-Mex Sausage

COOKING TIME: 12 MIN

DESCRIPTION

Delicious Tex-Mex sausage recipe that is spicy and hearty enough for a weekend's lazy brunch. The combo of spices and flavors really makes up for the low amount of sodium.

INGREDIENTS FOR 8 SERVINGS

- ½ pound of lean ground beef
- ¼ cup of white onion, thinly chopped
- 1 large clove of garlic, minced
- 1 tbsp of fresh cilantro, chopped
- 1 tbsp of vinegar
- 2 tbsp of canned green chilli peppers
- ¼ tsp salt
- 1 tsp of chilli powder

METHOD

1. In a mixing bowl, mix together cilantro, onions, green chilli peppers, garlic, vinegar, and chili powder.
2. Add the ground beef and mix again everything well.
3. Form the mixture into 8 equal flat or semi-flat patties.
4. Grease a skillet with a bit of vegetable oil. Place the patties on the pan over medium heat and let cook for 5-6 minutes on each side.

NUTRITIONAL INFORMATION (Per Serving)

- Calories: 88 kcal
- Carbohydrate: 1 g
- Protein: 11.58 g
- Sodium: 80 mg
- Potassium: 105 mg
- Phosphorus: 64 mg
- Dietary Fiber: 0.4 g
- Fat: 9 g

European Pancakes

COOKING TIME: 15-20 MIN

DESCRIPTION

European pancakes, most favored by the French and the Germans are thin and soft and make an excellent base for other dishes-both savory and sweet. If you are making these for breakfast, top them with some fresh strawberries and honey for a low potassium sweet treat.

INGREDIENTS FOR 10 SERVINGS

(20 pancakes)

- 2/3 cups of all-purpose flour

- 4 large eggs

- 2 tbsp of sugar

- ½ tsp of lemon zest

- 1 cup of low-fat milk

- ¼ tsp of vanilla extract

METHOD

1. In a medium bowl, mix together the flour with the sugar. Whisk in the eggs and combine well.
2. Add the milk, vanilla and lemon zest to the mix and whisk well.
3. Spray a small 8-10 inch pan with cooking spray and pour around 4 tbsp of the mixture and distribute evenly by tilting the pan from one side to another.
4. Cook until the batter is solid and light golden brown (around 50 seconds on each side). Flip.
5. Repeat the above two steps until all the batter has finished.
6. Serve.

NUTRITIONAL INFORMATION (Per Serving)

- Calories: 74 kcal
- Carbohydrate: 10 g

- Protein: 4 g
- Sodium: 39 mg
- Potassium: 73 mg
- Phosphorus: 73 mg
- Dietary Fiber: 0.2 g
- Fat: 2 g

Multigrain Warm Porridge

COOKING TIME: 30 MIN

DESCRIPTION

A hearty breakfast recipe that combines 3 types of low potassium grains along with oats for a nice contrast of flavors and textures. If you have 30 minutes to spare, you need to try this.

INGREDIENTS FOR 2 SERVINGS

- 2 cups of water
- 2 tbsp of old fashioned grits
- 1 tbsp of uncooked roasted buckwheat
- 1 tbsp of steel cut oats, uncooked
- 3 tbsp of plain couscous
- 1 tsp of honey
- 1 tsp of cinnamon

METHOD

1. Bring the water to boil in a small pot.
2. Add grits and stir for a few seconds.
3. Add the buckwheat and the oats, stir for a few seconds and lower the heat. Cover the pot and let simmer for 20 minutes.
4. Remove the lid from the pot and add the couscous. Take off the heat and let sit covered for another 5 minutes.
5. Transfer into a cereal bowl and sprinkle some honey and cinnamon or blueberries on top.

NUTRITIONAL INFORMATION (Per Serving)

- Calories: 298 kcal
- Carbohydrate: 60.3 g
- Protein: 9 g
- Sodium: 0.5 g
- Potassium: 78 mg
- Phosphorus: 25.2 mg
- Dietary Fiber: 3 g
- Fat: 1 g

Puffy French Toast

COOKING TIME: 8 MIN

DESCRIPTION

An easy French toast recipe that is dairy-free for lower amounts of phosphorus. Made in the pan and finished in the oven for an extra puffy result.

INGREDIENTS FOR 4 SERVINGS

- 4 slices of white bread, cut in half diagonally
- 3 whole eggs and 1 egg white
- 1 cup of plain almond milk
- 2 tbsp of canola oil
- 1 tsp of cinnamon

METHOD

1. Preheat your oven to 400F/180C
2. Beat together the eggs with the almond milk.

3. Heat the oil in a pan.

4. Dip each bread slice/triangle into the egg and almond milk mixture.

5. Fry in the pan until golden brown on each side.

6. Place the toasts in a baking dish and let cook in the oven for another 5 minutes.

7. Serve warm and drizzle with some honey, icing sugar, or cinnamon on top.

NUTRITIONAL INFORMATION (Per Serving)

- Calories: 293.75 kcal
- Carbohydrate: 25.3 g
- Protein: 9.27 g
- Sodium: 211 g
- Potassium: 97 mg
- Phosphorus: 165 mg
- Dietary Fiber: 12.3 g
- Fat: 16.50 g

Lunch

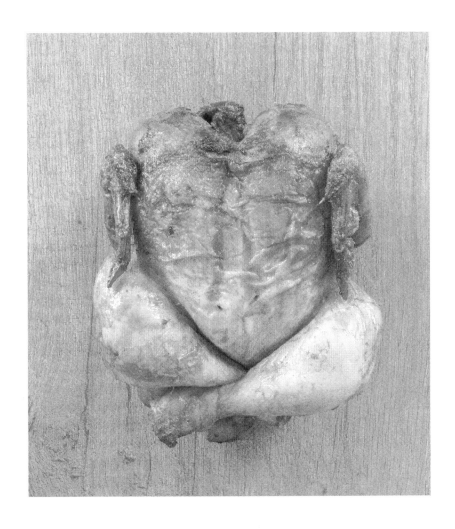

Couscous with Veggies

COOKING TIME: 10 MIN

DESCRIPTION

Couscous is favorite grain as it's very easy and quick to make. If you wish to have your daily dose of veggies in a more delicious and easy to eat way, try this recipe.

INGREDIENTS FOR 5 SERVINGS

- ½ cup of uncooked couscous
- ¼ cup of white mushrooms, sliced
- ½ cup of red onion, chopped
- 1 garlic clove, minced
- ½ cup of frozen peas
- 2 tbsp of dry white wine
- ½ tsp of basil
- 2 tbsp of fresh parsley, chopped
- 1 cup water or vegetable stock
- 1 tbsp of margarine or vegetable oil

METHOD

1. Thaw the peas by setting them aside at room temperature for 15-20 minutes.
2. In a medium pan, heat the margarine or vegetable oil.
3. Add the onions, peas, mushroom, and garlic and saute for around 5 minutes. Add the wine and let it evaporate.
4. Add all the herbs and spices and toss well. Take off the heat and keep aside.
5. In a small pot, cook the couscous with 1 cup of hot water or vegetable stock. Bring to a boil, take off the heat and let sit for a few minutes with a lid covered.
6. Add the saute veggies to the couscous and toss well.
7. Serve in a serving bowl warm or cold.

NUTRITIONAL INFORMATION (Per Serving)

- Calories: 110.4 kcal
- Carbohydrate: 18 g

- Protein: 3 g
- Sodium: 112.2 mg
- Potassium: 69.6 mg
- Phosphorus: 46.8 mg
- Dietary Fiber: 2.1 g
- Fat: 2 g

Mexican Steak Tacos

COOKING TIME: 15 MIN

DESCRIPTION

Tacos are a trademark dish of Mexican cuisine and if you wish to make them like Tex-Mex, here is a taco recipe with steak as the key ingredient.

INGREDIENTS FOR 8 SERVINGS.

- 1 pound of flank or skirt steak
- ¼ cup of fresh cilantro, chopped
- ¼ cup white onion, chopped
- 3 limes, juiced
- 3 cloves of garlic, minced
- 2 tsp of garlic powder
- 2 tbsp of olive oil
- ½ cup of Mexican or mozzarella cheese, grated
- 1 tsp of Mexican seasoning
- 8 medium-sized (6") corn flour tortillas.

METHOD

1. Combine the juice from two limes, Mexican seasoning and garlic powder in a dish or bowl and marinate the steak with it for at least half an hour in the fridge.

2. In a separate bowl, combine the chopped cilantro, garlic, onion and juice from one lime to make your salsa. Cover and keep in the fridge.

3. Heat the olive oil in a medium pan. Slice steak into thin strips and cook for approx. 3 minutes on each side.

4. Preheat your oven to 350F/180C.

5. Distribute evenly the steak strips in each tortilla. Top with a tablespoon of the grated cheese on top.

6. Wrap each taco in aluminum foil and bake in the oven for approx. 7-8 minutes or until cheese is melted.

7. Serve warm with your cilantro salsa.

NUTRITIONAL INFORMATION (Per Serving)

- Calories: 230 kcal
- Carbohydrate: 19.5 g
- Protein: 15 g
- Sodium: 486.75 g
- Potassium: 240 mg
- Phosphorus: 268 mg
- Dietary Fiber: 0.1 g
- Fat: 11 g

Beer Pork Ribs

COOKING TIME: 8 HOURS

DESCRIPTION

A juicy pork ribs recipe made with root beer and three other ingredients for minimal fuss. If you have a slow cooker and wish to have a delicious family meal for lunch, this is worth trying out.

INGREDIENTS FOR 6 SERVINGS.

- 2 pounds of pork ribs, cut in two units/racks
- 18 oz. of root beer
- 2 cloves of garlic, minced
- 2 tbsp of onion powder
- 2 tbsp of vegetable oil (optional)

METHOD

1. Wrap the pork ribs with vegetable oil and place one unit on the bottom of your slow

cooker with half of the minced garlic and the onion powder. Place the other rack on top with the rest of the garlic and onion powder.

2. Pour over the root beer and cover the lid.
3. Let simmer for 8 hours on low heat.
4. Take off and finish optionally in a grilling pan for a nice sear.

NUTRITIONAL INFORMATION (Per Serving)

- Calories: 301 kcal
- Carbohydrate: 36 g
- Protein: 21 g
- Sodium: 729 mg
- Potassium: 200 mg
- Phosphorus: 209 mg
- Dietary Fiber: 0 g
- Fat: 18 g

Crispy Lemon Chicken

COOKING TIME: 10 MIN

DESCRIPTION

This delicious lemon chicken recipe looks complex but it's actually very easy to cook. The breading also adds a nice crunch to its lemony sauce.

INGREDIENTS FOR 6 SERVINGS

- 1 pound of boneless and skinless, chicken breast
- ½ cup of all-purpose flour
- 1 large egg
- ½ cup of lemon juice
- 2 tbsp of water
- ¼ tsp salt
- ¼ tsp lemon pepper
- 1 tsp of mixed herb seasoning
- 2 tbsp of olive oil
- A few lemon slices for garnishing

65

- 1 tbsp of chopped parsley (for garnishing)
- 2 cups of cooked plain white rice

METHOD

1. Cut the chicken breast into thin slices and season with the herb seasoning, salt, and pepper.
2. In a small bowl, whisk together the egg with the water.
3. Keep the flour in a separate bowl.
4. Dip the chicken slices in the egg bath and then into the flour. Ensure that all sides are coated with flour.
5. Heat your oil in a medium frying pan.
6. Shallow fry the chicken in the pan until golden brown (approx. 3 minutes on each side).
7. Add the lemon juice and cook for another couple of minutes.

8. Taken the chicken out of the pan and transfer on a wide dish with absorbing paper to absorb any excess oil.

9. Garnish with some chopped parsley and lemon wedges on top and serve with the cooked white rice.

NUTRITIONAL INFORMATION (Per Serving)

- Calories: 232 kcal
- Carbohydrate: 24 g
- Protein: 18 g
- Sodium: 100 g
- Potassium: 234 mg
- Phosphorus: 217 mg
- Dietary Fiber: 0.8 g
- Fat: 8 g

Mexican Chorizo Sausage

COOKING TIME: 15 MIN

DESCRIPTION

A sausage patty enhanced with true Mexican and Spanish flavors that fans of mildly spicy food will love. Serve ideally with Mexican salsa and some roasted veggies.

INGREDIENTS FOR 16 SERVINGS.

- 2 pounds of boneless pork but, coarsely ground
- 3 tbsp of red wine vinegar
- 2 tbsp of smoked paprika
- ½ tsp of cinnamon
- ½ tsp of ground cloves
- ¼ tsp of coriander seeds
- ¼ tsp ground ginger
- 1 tsp of ground cumin
- 3 tbsp of brandy

METHOD

1. In a large mixing bowl, combine the ground pork with the seasonings, brandy, and vinegar and mix with your hands well.

2. Place the mixture into a large Ziploc bag and leave in the fridge overnight, for all the flavors to blend with each other and for lightly curing the sausage.

3. Form into 15-16 patties of equal size.

4. Heat the oil in a large pan and fry the patties for approx. 5-7 minutes on each side, or until the meat inside is no longer pink and there is a light brown crust on top.

5. Serve hot.

NUTRITIONAL INFORMATION (Per Serving)

- Calories: 134 kcal
- Carbohydrate: 0 g
- Protein: 10 g

- Sodium: 40 mg
- Potassium: 138 mg
- Phosphorus: 128 mg
- Dietary Fiber: 0 g
- Fat: 7 g

Eggplant Casserole

DESCRIPTION

Eggplant is one of these veggies that people either love or hate, but if you cook it along with other ingredients, as in this casserole recipe it makes an incredibly delicious meal for the entire family.

INGREDIENTS FOR 4 SERVINGS.

- 3 cups of eggplant, peeled and cut into large chunks
- 2 egg whites
- 1 large egg, whole
- ½ cup of unsweetened vegetable e.g. soy or almond cream
- ¼ tsp of sage
- ½ cup of breadcrumbs
- 1 tbsp of margarine, melted
- 1/4 tsp garlic salt

METHOD

1. Preheat the oven at 350F/180C.
2. Place the eggplants chunks in a medium pan, cover with a bit of water and let cook with the lid covered until tender. Drain from the water and mash with a tool or fork.
3. Beat the eggs with the non-dairy vegetable cream, sage, salt, and pepper. Whisk in the eggplant mush.
4. Combine the melted margarine with the breadcrumbs.
5. Bake in the oven for 20-25 minutes or until the casserole has a golden brown crust.

NUTRITIONAL INFORMATION (Per Serving)

- Calories: 186 kcal
- Carbohydrate: 19 g
- Protein: 7 g
- Sodium: 503 mg

- Potassium: 230 mg
- Phosphorus: 62 mg
- Dietary Fiber: 17.4 g
- Fat: 9 g

Easy Cilantro Cod

COOKING TIME: 8 MIN

DESCRIPTION

An incredibly easy recipe made with the fresh, sharp, and zesty flavors of lemon and cilantro. Make this with cod preferably but feel free to substitute with tilapia or haddock.

INGREDIENTS FOR 4 SERVINGS

- 1 pound of cod fillets, at room temperature
- ½ cup of mayonnaise
- ½ cup of fresh cilantro, chopped
- 2 tbsp of lime juice

METHOD

1. In a mixing bowl, mix the mayo with the cilantro and lime juice. Keep a ¼ cup in a small bowl as a sauce to serve with the cod later.

2. Brush the remaining mayo mix on the fish.

3. Heat a bit of oil in a shallow big pan over medium heat. Add the cod fillets and cook for approx. 3-4 minutes on each side.

4. Serve with the reserved cilantro and mayo sauce.

NUTRITIONAL INFORMATION (Per Serving)

- Calories: 322 kcal
- Carbohydrate: 1 g
- Protein: 26 g
- Sodium: 612 g
- Potassium: 237 mg
- Phosphorus: 218 mg
- Dietary Fiber: 0 g
- Fat: 23 g

Light Greek Soutzoukakia

COOKING TIME: 30 MIN

DESCRIPTION

"Soutzoukakia" is Greek/Turkish meatballs that are passed along many generations of Greeks and are renowned for the spicy and aromatic taste. Here is a lighter version of the original recipe.

INGREDIENTS FOR 8-10 SERVINGS

- 1 pound of ground beef (around 90% lean)
- 2 tbsp of red wine
- 1 tbsp of cumin
- 1 tsp of cinnamon
- ½ tsp of nutmeg
- ½ tsp of black pepper
- 2 tbsp of bread crumbs
- 1 large egg white
- ½ cup of tomato sauce

- Olive oil

METHOD

1. Preheat the oven at 350F/180C.
2. Mix all the ingredients in a mixing bowl.
3. Grease your hands and a baking tray with a bit of olive oil. Shape with your greased hands into small yet elongated meatballs (around 20-25 in pieces in total).
4. Bake in the oven for 30 minutes.
5. Heat the ready-made tomato sauce for 5 minutes and pour over the Soutzoukakia.

NUTRITIONAL INFORMATION (Per Serving)

- Calories: 174 kcal
- Carbohydrate: 8.1 g
- Protein: 19.8 g
- Sodium: 126 mg
- Potassium: 200 mg
- Phosphorus: 95.5 mg
- Dietary Fiber: 1.2 g
- Fat: 8.8 g

Pizza with Chicken & Pesto

COOKING TIME: 25 MIN

DESCRIPTION

This low potassium pizza recipe is easy to make and has a burst of flavors. Try it with chicken and pesto, that blends ideally Italian and American flavors.

INGREDIENTS FOR 4 SERVINGS

- 1 ready-made frozen pizza dough
- ⅔ cup cooked chicken, chopped
- ½ cup of orange bell pepper, diced
- ½ cup of green bell pepper, diced
- ¼ cup of purple onion, chopped
- 2 tbsp of green basil pesto
- 1 tbsp of chives, chopped
- ⅓ cup of parmesan or Romano cheese, grated
- ¼ cup of mozzarella cheese
- 1 tbsp of olive oil

METHOD

1. Thaw the pizza dough according to instructions on the package.
2. Heat the olive oil in a pan and saute the peppers and onions for a couple of minutes. Set aside
3. Once the pizza dough has thawed, spread the bali pesto over its surface.
4. Top with half of the cheese, the peppers, the onions, and the chicken. Finish with the rest of the cheese.
5. Bake at 350F/180C for approx. 20 minutes (or until crust and cheese are baked).
6. Slice in triangles with a pizza cutter or sharp knife and serve.

NUTRITIONAL INFORMATION (Per Serving)

- Calories: 225 kcal
- Carbohydrate: 13.9 g
- Protein: 11.1 g

- Sodium: 321 mg
- Potassium: 174 mg
- Phosphorus: 172 mg
- Dietary Fiber: 1.2 g
- Fat: 12 g

Easy Egg Salad

COOKING TIME: 8 MIN

DESCRIPTION

A quick and easy version of the old-school egg salad recipe that is perfect for making ahead of school or work lunch. Combine ideally in lettuce wraps or white bread as a sandwich filling.

INGREDIENTS FOR 4 SERVINGS

- 4 large eggs
- ½ cup of sweet onion, chopped
- ¼ cup of celery, chopped
- 2 tbsp of pickle relish
- 1 tbsp of yellow mustard
- 1 tsp of smoked paprika
- 3 tbsp of mayo

METHOD

1. Hard boil the eggs in a small pot filled with water for approx. 7-8 minutes. Leave

the eggs in the water for an extra couple of minutes before peeling.

2. Peel the eggs and chop finely with a knife or tool.

3. Combine all the chopped veggies with the mayo and mustard. Add in the eggs and mix well.

4. Sprinkle with some smoked paprika on top.

5. Serve cold with pitta, white bread slices, or lettuce wraps.

NUTRITIONAL INFORMATION (Per Serving)

- Calories: 127 kcal
- Carbohydrate: 6 g
- Protein: 7 g
- Sodium: 170.7 mg
- Potassium: 87.5 mg
- Phosphorus: 101 mg
- Dietary Fiber: 0.17 g
- Fat: 13 g

Shrimp Quesadilla

COOKING TIME: 10 MIN

DESCRIPTION

Quesadilla is a favorite Tex-Mex lunch for kids and you can make it for lunch using two corn flour tortillas and filled with a nice blend of shrimps, peppers, and cheese inside.

INGREDIENTS FOR 2 SERVINGS

- 5 oz of shrimp, shelled and deveined
- 4 tbsp of Mexican salsa
- 2 tbsp of fresh cilantro, chopped
- 1 tbsp of lemon juice
- 1 tsp of ground cumin
- 1 tsp of cayenne pepper
- 2 tbsp of unsweetened soy yogurt or creamy tofu
- 2 medium corn flour tortillas
- 2 tbsp of low-fat cheddar cheese

METHOD

1. Mix the cilantro, cumin, lemon juice, and the cayenne in a Ziploc bag to make your marinade. Add the shrimps and marinade for 10 minutes.
2. Heat a pan over medium heat with some olive oil and toss in the shrimp with the marinade. Let cook for a couple of minutes or as soon as shrimps have turned pink and opaque.
3. Add the soy cream or soft tofu in the pan and mix well. Remove from the heat and keep the marinade aside.
4. Heat tortillas in the grill or microwave for a few seconds.
5. Place 2 tbsp of salsa on each tortilla. Top one tortilla with the shrimp mixture and add the cheese on top.
6. Stack one tortilla against each other (with the spread salsa layer facing the shrimp mixture).

7. Transfer this on a baking tray and cook for 7-8 minutes at 350F/180C to melt the cheese and crisp up the tortillas.
8. Serve warm.

NUTRITIONAL INFORMATION (Per Serving)

- Calories: 255 kcal
- Carbohydrate: 21 g
- Protein: 24 g
- Sodium: 562 g
- Potassium: 235 mg
- Phosphorus: 189 mg
- Dietary Fiber: 2 g
- Fat: 9 g

Grilled Corn on the Cob

COOKING TIME: 20 MIN

DESCRIPTION

A barbeque favorite for vegans and meat-eaters alike that instantly brightens your mood and satisfy your appetite.

INGREDIENTS FOR 4 SERVINGS

- 4 frozen corn on the cob, cut in half
- ½ tsp of thyme
- 1 tbsp of grated parmesan cheese
- ¼ tsp of black pepper

METHOD

1. Combine the oil, cheese, thyme, and black pepper in a bowl.
2. Place the corn in the cheese/oil mix and roll to coat evenly.
3. Fold all 4 pieces in aluminum foil, leaving a small open surface on top.

4. Place the wrapped corns over the grill and let cook for 20 minutes.

NUTRITIONAL INFORMATION (Per Serving)

- Calories: 125 kcal
- Carbohydrate: 29.5 g
- Protein: 2 g
- Sodium: 26 g
- Potassium: 145 mg
- Phosphorus: 91.5 mg
- Dietary Fiber: 3.5 g
- Fat: 1.3 g

Dinner

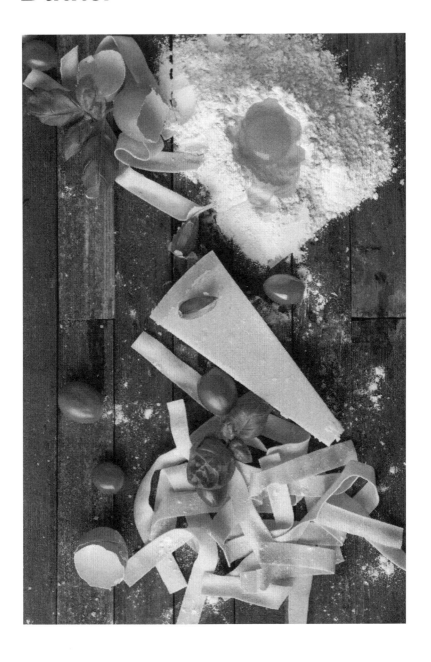

Creamy Crab Soup

COOKING TIME: 15-20 MIN

DESCRIPTION

An awesome soup recipe just like its name denotes - creamy and crabby. This recipe is close to the traditional Maryland eastern shore recipe but with lower potassium ingredients. Great as a family dinner for everyone.

INGREDIENTS FOR 7-8 SERVINGS

- 1 tbsp low salt butter
- 1 cup of white onion, chopped
- ½ pound of fresh crab meat
- 4 cups low salt chicken broth
- 1 cup of soy or vegetable cream
- 2 tbsp cornstarch
- ⅛ tsp dill
- Kosher pepper

METHOD

1. Melt the butter in a large pan over medium heat.
2. Add the onion to the pot and saute until transparent, for around 3 minutes.
3. Add the crab meat to the mix and cook for another couple of minutes.
4. Add the chicken broth to the pan mix and bring to a boil.
5. Mix the vegetable or soy cream with the cornstarch and whisk to combine well. Add to the soup and increase the heat to medium-high.
6. Add the dill and pepper and stir frequently until soup comes to a boil.
7. Serve hot.

NUTRITIONAL INFORMATION (Per Serving)

- Calories: 89 kcal
- Carbohydrate: 10 g
- Protein: 7 g
- Sodium: 228 mg
- Potassium: 237 mg

- Phosphorus: 83 mg
- Dietary Fiber: 0.3 g
- Fat: 3.7 g

Broccoli Onion Latkes

COOKING TIME: 10 MIN

DESCRIPTION

A tasty Jewish "latke" recipe with broccoli and onions that you can make in under 10 minutes.

INGREDIENTS FOR 4 SERVINGS

- 3 cups of broccoli florets, roughly chopped
- ½ cup of onion, thinly chopped
- 2 egg whites
- 2 tbsp of all-purpose flour
- 1 tsp of garlic salt
- 2 tbsp of olive oil

METHOD

1. Boil the broccoli in a pot covered with vegetable stock for 5 minutes or until tender.

2. Drain the broccoli and keep aside. Whisk eggs in a separate bowl and add the flour stirring well.

3. Add the onion into the flour and egg mixture. Add the drained broccoli and combine well.

4. Heat the olive oil in a shallow pan. Drop the mixture with a spoon and flatten with a spatula to make a patty.

5. Shallow fry until golden brown (2 minutes on each side) over medium heat.

6. Place on a dish with absorbing paper and serve hot.

NUTRITIONAL INFORMATION (Per Serving)

- Calories: 110 kcal
- Carbohydrate: 7.2 g
- Protein: 2.9 g
- Sodium: 204 mg
- Potassium: 162 mg
- Phosphorus: 46 mg

- Dietary Fiber: 1.96 g
- Fat: 7 g

Glazed Carrots

COOKING TIME: 25 MIN

DESCRIPTION

An easy recipe with carrots that you can make as a quick dinner or as a low potassium side dish for rice or meat. Great if you are a vegan as well.

INGREDIENTS FOR 4 SERVINGS

- 2 cups of carrots, sliced into 1'' slices
- 1 tbsp of white sugar
- 1 tsp of cornstarch
- 2 tbsp of margarine or vegetable shortening, melted
- ⅛ tsp of salt
- ¼ tsp of ground ginger
- ¼ cup of apple juice

METHOD

1. Poach the carrots in a pan filled with a ¼ cup of boiling water. Cook covered over medium heat until tender (around 12-15 minutes).
2. Combine together the sugar, corn starch, ginger, and salt. Add the melted margarine and apple juice and whisk well. Pour the mixture over the carrots in the pan with the water.
3. Allow cooking for around 8-10 minutes or until sauce thickens.

NUTRITIONAL INFORMATION (Per Serving)

- Calories: 101 kcal
- Carbohydrate: 14 g
- Protein: 1 g
- Sodium: 378 g
- Potassium: 202 mg
- Phosphorus: 22.7 mg
- Dietary Fiber: 2.7 g
- Fat: 5 g

Slow Cooker Chicken

COOKING TIME: 8 HOURS

DESCRIPTION

If you wish to have some chicken for a family, dinner this slow cooker recipe with just 5 ingredients is all you need. You can also use any leftovers for sandwiches or salads later.

INGREDIENTS FOR 8-9 SERVINGS

- 4 oz. of a whole chicken (uncut)
- 1 tbsp of all-purpose or chicken seasoning
- ½ tsp of black pepper
- ½ tsp of garlic powder
- 3 tbsp of wine

METHOD

1. Wash the chicken and remove any insides.

2. Wrap with the chicken seasoning, garlic powder, and pepper.
3. Place in a lightly greased slow cooker/crock-pot, add the wine and cover with the lid and set to low heat for 8 hours.
4. Remove the skin, cut and serve.

NUTRITIONAL INFORMATION (Per Serving)

- Calories: 131 kcal
- Carbohydrate: 0 g
- Protein: 7 g
- Sodium: 60 mg
- Potassium: 160 mg
- Phosphorus: 130 mg
- Dietary Fiber: 0 g
- Fat: 6 g

Syrian Style Lamb Kafta

COOKING TIME: 18-20 MIN

DESCRIPTION

Kafta is a traditional middle eastern lamb dish with spices that is best made on the charcoal grill, however, you can also make this in the oven's grill for convenience reasons. Serve ideally with chopped cucumber and tomatoes.

INGREDIENTS FOR 6 SERVINGS

- 1 pound of finely ground lamb
- 1 tsp of cumin
- 1 tsp of paprika
- 1 tsp of sumac or lemon pepper
- 2 cloves of garlic, minced
- 3 tbsp of chopped parsley
- 1 tbsp of olive oil
- ½ tsp of salt

METHOD

1. Combine all the ingredients together and mix well with your hands.
2. Preheat your oven's broiler.
3. Take 6 medium wooden sticks (for skewers) and wrap each with approx. 2 inches of the mixture.
4. Cook over a baking sheet for approx. 8-10 minutes on each side.

NUTRITIONAL INFORMATION (Per Serving)

- Calories: 170 kcal
- Carbohydrate: 0.8 g
- Protein: 13.5 g
- Sodium: 45 mg
- Potassium: 215 mg
- Phosphorus: 147 mg
- Dietary Fiber: 0.5 g
- Fat: 11.7 g

Spicy Lime Shrimp

COOKING TIME: 5 MIN

DESCRIPTION

A spicy and tangy shrimp recipe inspired by the Creole seafood flavors of New Orleans. If you are a fan of peppers and lime, you'll love this one.

INGREDIENTS FOR 4-5 SERVINGS

- 32 large shrimp, peeled and deveined
- ¼ cup of lime juice
- 1 garlic clove, minced
- 1 green onion, sliced
- 3 tbsp of red bell pepper, diced
- 2 tbsp of fresh cilantro, chopped
- 1 tsp of jalapeno chili, minced
- ⅛ tsp of salt
- 1 big cucumber, sliced

METHOD

1. To make your dressing, combine together the lime juice, green onion, jalapeno chili, cilantro, garlic, and oil or salt in a mixing bowl.

2. In a separate mixing bowl, add the shrimps with 3 tbsp of the lime juice marinade. Cover and let in the fridge for 40 minutes.

3. Turn on your oven's broiler. Discard the shrimp from the lime marinade and broil for around 3-4 minutes in total or 2 minutes on each side.

4. Take off the heat and pour the remaining marinade on top.

5. Place over the cucumber slices and serve cold.

NUTRITIONAL INFORMATION (Per Serving)

- Calories: 132 kcal
- Carbohydrate: 3 g
- Protein: 12 g
- Sodium: 149 mg

- Potassium: 202 mg
- Phosphorus: 128 mg
- Dietary Fiber: 0.6 g
- Fat: 8 g

Pasta Shells with Peas and Bacon

COOKING TIME: 12 MIN

DESCRIPTION

If you are a fan of comfort and rich flavors, this pasta dish with bacon, cream and peas will definitely become a favorite. The addition of parmesan cheese and butter makes it extra fragrant, without increasing much its potassium levels.

INGREDIENTS FOR 6 SERVINGS

- 1 cup of whole wheat pasta shells (you may also use penne pasta)
- ¾ cup of frozen peas
- 2 tbsp of unsalted butter
- ½ cup of parmesan cheese, grated
- 3 slices of bacon,
- 1 cup of white onion, chopped
- 2-3 cloves of garlic, minced

- ¼ tsp of kosher pepper
- 1 tbsp of lemon juice

METHOD

1. Boil the pasta into a pot filled with 1 liter of boiling water for 8-10 minutes (or according to packaging instructions). Add the peas during the last two minutes of cooking. Drain and keep the water aside.

2. Cut the butter with a knife into small chunks. Combine the ricotta and parmesan cheese in a separate big bowl to mix with pasta later.

3. Cut the bacon into thin strips and heat a skillet with cooking spray. Shallow fry until nice and crisp but not burned (around 6 minutes). Remove and set aside.

4. Add the onion to the same pan and cook until transparent, for approx. 3 minutes.

5. Add the minced garlic and saute for another minute. Transfer the onion and bacon mixture to cheese bowl.

6. Add ½ cup of the cooking water kept and the lemon juice to the cheese mixture. Add the drained pasta with the peas and toss to coat evenly.

7. Finish with the cooked bacon strips and some pepper to taste.

8. Serve warm.

NUTRITIONAL INFORMATION (Per Serving)

- Calories: 313 kcal
- Carbohydrate: 27 g
- Protein: 13 g
- Sodium: 244 g
- Potassium: 172 mg
- Phosphorus: 203 mg
- Dietary Fiber: 3.3 g
- Fat: 14 g

Buffalo Chicken Wings

COOKING TIME: 35 MIN

DESCRIPTION

An all-American dish, buffalo chicken wings are a famous dinner and side dish in football and festive nights. And the best part is that each counts only 105 mg of potassium per serving so feel free to eat as much as 5 wings.

INGREDIENTS FOR 12 SERVINGS

- 24 chicken wings (drumettes)

- ¼ cup of low sodium tomato sauce

- 8 tbsp of unsalted butter,

- ⅓ cup of hot pepper sauce e.g. Tabasco

- ½ tsp of garlic

- 1 tbsp of olive oil

- ½ tsp of Italian seasoning mix

- ¼ cup roasted red bell pepper puree/sauce.

METHOD

1. Preheat your oven 400F/190C.
2. Melt your butter in a pan.
3. Pour in the hot pepper sauce, the tomato sauce, garlic powder, olive oil, and Italian seasoning. Mix well with a spatula. Let heat for 2 minutes and remove from the heat.
4. Arrange the chicken wings on a baking sheet.
5. Brush the sauce over the chicken wings, making sure they are evenly coated and bake for 30-35 minutes.

NUTRITIONAL INFORMATION (Per Serving)

- Calories: 131 kcal
- Carbohydrate: 0.1 g
- Protein: 8 g

- Sodium: 64 mg
- Potassium: 105 mg
- Phosphorus: 61 mg
- Dietary Fiber: 0 g
- Fat: 11 g

Cauliflower and Apple Soup

COOKING TIME: 40 MIN

DESCRIPTION

A delicious vegetarian soup that blends ideally the flavors of cauliflower and apples with herbs and bread crostini as an optional addition on top. Perfect for family weekend dinner.

INGREDIENTS FOR 12 SERVINGS

- 1 head of cauliflower, chopped into small chunks
- 1 cup of white onion, diced
- 1 cup of apple, thinly cubed
- 2 cloves of garlic, minced
- 6 cups of chicken stock
- 1 tsp of thyme,
- 1 tsp of rosemary
- 1 tsp of sage
- 12 baguette slices
- 1 tbsp of garlic powder

METHOD

1. To make the bread and garlic crostini, drizzle the baguette slices with olive oil, the minced garlic and the garlic powder. Bake in a preheated oven at 350F/175C for 10 minutes. Keep aside.

2. To make the soup, bring the chicken stock to a boil and add the vegetables, the apple, and the rest ingredients. Let cook with the lid covered for 25-30 minutes.

3. Transfer the soup in a deep soup dish and blend with a hand immersion blender.

4. Serve in individual soup bowls with some sliced bread crostini on top.

NUTRITIONAL INFORMATION (Per Serving)

- Calories: 82 kcal
- Carbohydrate: 15 g
- Protein: 3 g

- Sodium: 125 mg
- Potassium: 231 mg
- Phosphorus: 64 mg
- Dietary Fiber: 2 g
- Fat: 1.1 g

Mapo's Tofu and Pork

COOKING TIME: 15 MIN

DESCRIPTION

A traditional Chinese dish with tofu and pork as the main ingredients with a spicy and slightly oily sauce. You can make it with shrimps or chicken in place of the pork if you wish.

INGREDIENTS FOR 8 SERVINGS.

- 3 oz/120 gr of ground pork
- 1 block (350gr) medium firm tofu
- 2 cloves of garlic, minced
- 1 tsp of red chilli flakes
- 1 green onion, sliced

For the marinade:

- 1 tbsp of sesame oil
- 1 tsp of low sodium soy sauce
- 1 tsp rice vinegar or dry white wine
- 1 tbsp of vegetable oil

- ½ tsp of white sugar

For the sauce:

- 1/s tsp low sodium sauce
- 1 tsp of sesame oil
- 3 tbsp of water
- 1 tbsp of cornstarch

METHOD

1. Mix together all the marinade ingredients in a bowl. Add the pork and allow to marinate for approx. 15 minutes.
2. Mix all the sauce ingredients in a separate bowl and keep aside.
3. Heat the vegetable oil in a wok or skillet and saute the garlic with the chilli flakes. Add the pork and stir-fry until fully cooked and no longer pink.
4. Add the tofu and stir gently to mix with the rest of the ingredients.

5. Stir in the sauce mix and stir repeatedly until it thickens.

6. Garnish optionally with a few spring onion slices.

7. Serve warm.

NUTRITIONAL INFORMATION (Per Serving)

- Calories: 110 kcal
- Carbohydrate: 3.3 g
- Protein: 7.4 g
- Sodium: 35 mg
- Potassium: 102 mg
- Phosphorus: 68 mg
- Dietary Fiber: 0.7 g
- Fat: 8.5 g

Lemon Orzo Salad

COOKING TIME: 10 MIN

DESCRIPTION

A lovely pasta salad with lemon, orzo and other herbs that is perfect for spring or summer evenings with friends or family. Great as next day much at work too.

INGREDIENTS FOR 4 SERVINGS

- 1 cup of orzo pasta
- 1 tsp of chicken bouillon granules
- 1 green onion, diced
- 1 red bell pepper, diced
- 2 tbsp of tarragon, chopped
- 2 tbsp of fresh parsley leaves, chopped
- 1 clove of garlic, minced
- 2 tbsp of lemon juice
- 1 tbsp of olive oil

METHOD

1. Cook the orzo in 3 cups of boiling water with the bouillon granules dissolved for 10-12 minutes (or based on package instructions).
2. Rinse with cold water and drain. Keep aside.
3. Add the rest of the ingredients in a salad bowl, toss to combine well and serve cool.

NUTRITIONAL INFORMATION (Per Serving)

- Calories: 148 kcal
- Carbohydrate: 24 g
- Protein: 4 g
- Sodium: 7 mg
- Potassium: 164 mg
- Phosphorus: 65 mg
- Dietary Fiber: 1.6 g
- Fat: 4 g

Sausage Stuffed Jalapenos

COOKING TIME: 20 MIN

DESCRIPTION

Delicious dinner recipe with ground pork sausage, cheese, and spices as the filling for roasted jalapeno boats.

INGREDIENTS FOR 12 SERVINGS.

- 1 pound of ground pork sausage
- 1 oz. of low fat and softened cream cheese
- 1 cup of ranch dressing (optional)
- 1 cup of parmesan cheese, grated

METHOD

1. Preheat the oven at 400F/190C.
2. Place the ground sausage in a skillet over medium heat and cook until brown. Drain and set aside.

3. Combine the sausage, cream cheese, and parmesan cheese in a mixing bowl.
4. Fill the jalapeno halves with approx.1 tbsp of the mixture each.
5. Place over a baking sheet and bake in the oven for 20 minutes.

NUTRITIONAL INFORMATION (Per Serving)

- Calories: 362 kcal
- Carbohydrate: 4.3 g
- Protein: 9.2 g
- Sodium: 601 mg
- Potassium: 199 mg
- Phosphorus: 68 mg
- Dietary Fiber: 1.1 g
- Fat: 34.2 g

Dessert

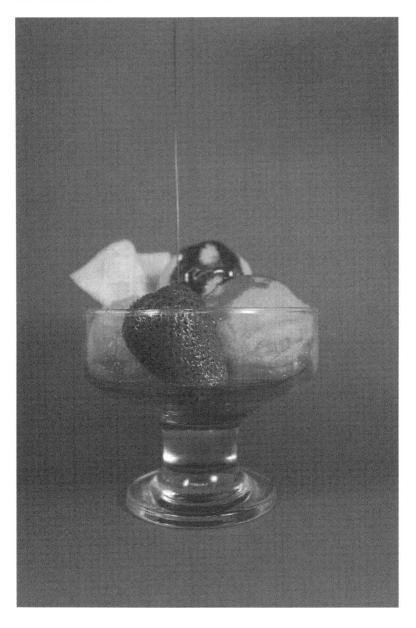

Raspberry Mousse

COOKING TIME: 12 MIN

DESCRIPTION

An easy, light and fruity raspberry mousse recipe that is perfect for a spring or summer dessert.

INGREDIENTS FOR 6 SERVINGS.

- 1 cup of frozen raspberries
- ¼ cup of water
- 2 tbsp of no sugar added jelly powder
- 1 ½ cup of whipping cream
- 1 pack of fresh raspberries

METHOD

1. Place the raspberries in a pot filled with the water. Cook until raspberries have softened (around 10-12 minutes).
2. Transfer the mixture in a bowl. Add the jelly powder and stir well to dissolve.

3. Once the mixture has cooled down, add in the whipping cream. Distribute the mixture into 6 dessert bowls or glasses.
4. Chill for at least a couple of hours prior serving.
5. Garnish with a tbsp of fresh raspberries on top of each serving.

NUTRITIONAL INFORMATION (Per Serving)

- Calories: 94 kcal
- Carbohydrate: 20.1 g
- Protein: 1.1 g
- Sodium: 22 mg
- Potassium: 133 mg
- Phosphorus: 28 mg
- Dietary Fiber: 5.2 g
- Fat: 1.61 g

Honey Ginger Cookies

COOKING TIME: 10 MIN

DESCRIPTION

A lovely cookie recipe with ginger if you wish to bake something fast and enjoy with your afternoon coffee or tea. You can also keep these up to two weeks.

INGREDIENTS FOR 15 SERVINGS

(30 cookies)

- 2 cups of all-purpose flour
- ¾ cups of vegetable shortening
- 1 cup of white sugar
- ¼ cup honey
- 2 tsp of baking soda
- 1 tsp of ginger powder
- 1 ¼ tsp of cinnamon
- 1 tsp of ground cloves
- A bit of icing sugar (for the top)

METHOD

1. Preheat the oven to 325 F/175C.
2. Combine all the cream/wet ingredients in a mixing bowl and beat well.
3. In a separate bowl, sift the flour and combine with the sugar and all the other ingredients.
4. Add the wet ingredients into the dry mixture and mix fast and well.
5. Roll into balls with your hands and place over a greased paper sheet, making sure each cookie ball is at least 1 inch apart from the other.
6. Bake for 8-10 minutes.

NUTRITIONAL INFORMATION (Per Serving)

- Calories: 112 kcal
- Carbohydrate: 16 g
- Protein: 1 g
- Sodium: 90 mg
- Potassium: 18 mg

- Phosphorus: 13 mg
- Dietary Fiber: 0.4 g
- Fat: 5 g

Honey Baked Pear

COOKING TIME: 30 MIN

DESCRIPTION

A nice alternative version to classic poached pear recipe, baked in the oven and enhanced with 5 spices for extra aroma and flavor.

INGREDIENTS FOR 8 SERVINGS.

- 4 pears, peeled and halved
- ¼ cup of unsalted butter or margarine
- ¼ cup of lemon juice
- ½ tsp of 5-spice powder
- 1 tsp of orange zest
- 1 tsp of vanilla extract

METHOD

1. Preheat the oven at 350F/175C.
2. Pour the lemon juice over the pears to avoid any darkening.

3. Mix the melted butter, spices, zest and vanilla in a bowl. Pour over the pears.
4. Place the marinated pears in an oven-safe pan and bake for 25-30 minutes.
5. Serve warm.

NUTRITIONAL INFORMATION (Per Serving)

- Calories: 141 kcal
- Carbohydrate: 23 g
- Protein: 0.5 g
- Sodium: 2 mg
- Potassium: 121 mg
- Phosphorus: 12 mg
- Dietary Fiber: 2.7 g
- Fat: 6 g

Watermelon Sorbet

COOKING TIME: 1 MIN

DESCRIPTION

Refreshing and cooling sorbet recipe that is perfect for chilling during hot summer days (and nights). It has only 52 calories per serving so no need to worry about ruining your weight loss diet.

INGREDIENTS FOR 2 SERVINGS

- 1 cup of ice, crushed
- 1 cup of watermelon chunks, seeded
- 2 tbsp of lime juice
- 1 tbsp of sugar
- 2 small watermelon slices (for garnishing)

METHOD

1. Pulse all the ingredients except for the watermelon slices in a blender for 30 seconds to 1 minute.

2. Pour the mixture into 2 mason jars or glasses, top with the wedges and serve chilled immediately.

NUTRITIONAL INFORMATION (Per Serving)

- Calories: 52 kcal
- Carbohydrate: 13 g
- Protein: 0 g
- Sodium: 1 mg
- Potassium: 96 mg
- Phosphorus: 9 mg
- Dietary Fiber: 0.3 g
- Fat: 0 g

Aunt Tula's Carrot Cake

COOKING TIME: 50 MIN

DESCRIPTION

A recipe close to the traditional old school carrot cake recipe with a bit of a twist. Make it and serve with your daily coffee or tea. Good for ladies' parties as well.

INGREDIENTS FOR 20 SERVINGS.

- 2 cups all-purpose flour
- 1 cup of white sugar
- 3 cups of carrot
- 1 cup of vegetable oil
- 4 large eggs, beaten
- 2 tbsp of skimmed milk
- 8 oz. of cream cheese
- ¼ cup unsalted butter
- 2 tsp of cinnamon
- 1 tsp of vanilla extract
- 2 tsp vanilla powder

- 1 cup of icing sugar

METHOD

1. Preheat the oven at 350F/180C.
2. In a large mixing bowl, combine all the dry ingredients e.g. flour, sugar, and others. Slowly incorporate the oil, the beaten eggs, the vanilla, and the milk. Mix well until mixture is uniform and slightly fluffy.
3. Pour the cake batter onto a lightly greased cake pan (around 9x11 inches)
4. Bake for 45-50 minutes
5. In a separate mixing bowl, beat the cream cheese with the icing sugar and vanilla powder to make your frosting.
6. Spread over the cooled carrot cake with a flat spatula. Slice and serve.

NUTRITIONAL INFORMATION (Per Serving)

- Calories: 324 kcal

- Carbohydrate: 34 g
- Protein: 4 g
- Sodium: 180.7 mg
- Potassium: 98 mg
- Phosphorus: 54 mg
- Dietary Fiber: 1 g
- Fat: 19 g

Conclusion

As specified earlier, while we have made an effort to include in this Renal Diet Cookbook recipes that are low in potassium, sodium, and phosphorus, it's best to consult with your doctor or nutritionist when trying out new recipes to confirm that the amounts and limits of the above key nutrients are suitable for your renal damage stage. Those that are currently on an earlier stage of CKD, for example, may consume up to 2000 mg of potassium per day, throughout their daily meals, which is a relatively easy target, considering that the average person consumes around 2500 mg of potassium or less per day. Respectively, the total daily intake of phosphorus should not surpass 600 mg (per day) but since most recipes contain less than 150 mg of phosphorus, this target isn't hard to achieve. Finally, the daily limit of sodium for renal patients with potential diabetes and/or heart disease should be up to 1500 mg/day.

If you know exactly the nutritional info for each recipe, as in the case of this book, it's also recommended to keep a journal of the meals/recipes you consume per day and show it to your doctor so you can both track your diet habits better.

Please always consult with your family doctor or nutritionist before using a current recipe or the diet program.

Thanks for your attention!

Written by: Albert Simon
Copyright © 2019.
All rights reserved.

Made in the USA
Monee, IL
25 February 2020